Behold this
HEART
in the Season of
ADVENT

A CANCER JOURNEY
WITH JESUS AND MARY

ALICE SEIDEL

Behold, This Heart in the Season of Advent

A Cancer Journey With Jesus and Mary by Alice Seidel

Copyright © 2019 Alice Seidel

Cover Design by 100Covers.com
Interior Design by FormattedBooks.com

1972seidel@gmail.com

To my loving husband Bob,
My children
Stephanie, Rob & Lisa
and
My beautiful grand daughters
Julia & Marisa

"For I know the plans I have for you, says the Lord, plans for welfare and not for evil, to give you a future and a hope."

Jeremiah 29:11

CONTENTS

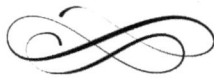

INTRODUCTION

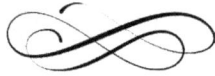

You have cancer.

He might as well have said, "you died yesterday, what are you doing here?"

Me? Not me. Are you kidding me!

It was stunning to hear those words falling from the mouth of the urologist. I don't get cancer, I don't want cancer. How will I rid myself of this curse? I don't know anything at all about it, and where do I even begin.

Because to my mind, cancer has always been a death sentence. Yes, people have it, had it, survive it, get it again, and lose it again, but inevitably it all catches up with you. Will it be a year, three years, five years, next month? Just what am I supposed to do?

I recall starting this book on the Wednesday of Epiphany week.

Epiphany. That long-forgotten feast that comes on January 6th. The one which practically no one remembers anymore. It can only be rivaled by its predecessor, Advent.

Advent. That quiet season.

Or so I used to think. Because after 67 years, Advent has been transformed for me. So, let me tell you all about it. That is the intent of this little book; to take a look back at all that was, and to connect it to my favorite liturgical season, Advent.

The weekend of the 21st of July 2018 had been such a nice one. One of my nieces, Karen, was having her bridal shower and myself, my daughter Stephanie, my daughter-in-law Lisa and my grand-daughters Julia and Marisa were going. We picked up my sister-in-law Diane and away we went to Staten Island. The shower was held outdoors, in the backyard and the decorations looked beautiful! We had such a nice time and I was truly looking forward to the wedding in September.

We were able to enjoy that afternoon and it was so good to be surrounded by family and meet the friends of my niece, Karen. I didn't have a clue to what was coming and to what was already wreaking havoc internally. Sometimes you have to thank God for not having foresight.

Have you ever been awakened in the middle of the night with a pain in your side or back? On Tuesday morning about 2:00 a.m., on July 24th, it happened to me. I was awakened by a pain in my back. I thought it was just from sleeping funny. It seemed to be in my right kidney. So, I turned over figuring the pain would just go away.

It didn't. And it continued to get worse.

By 5:00 a.m. I was laying sideways on the living room couch dozing slightly. The pain would ebb then flow back again as painful as ever. Eventually I got dressed and even tried to do some article writing (I'm a freelance writer) which was due back in a few days. I had to abandon that idea as the pain in my kidney got worse and worse.

By 10 o'clock or so, I texted my husband, Bob, who was working four hours a day, four days a week. I told him, please come home now, I have to go to the Urgent Care or somewhere. Then I got the bright idea to take some Tylenol; perhaps that would kill the pain.

One minute after swallowing those painkillers, they came right back up. I figured this must be a kidney stone; something I've never had ever in my life. By the time Bob walked in I was writhing in pain on the recliner in the back room. He called an ambulance. I couldn't believe this was happening.

I was in good health. Nothing was wrong, aside from some seasonal allergies. What was going on!

Long story short, a CT scan at the ER revealed a 'nodule or mass' (to quote the ER doctor) in my bladder. The take-home paperwork indicated this was most likely a 'neo-plasm' of some kind. Having been a medical records person for some years at a local nursing home in the 1980s - 90s, I knew the word 'neo-plasm' meant cancer. How could this be happening!

A week later I had a TURBT, or bladder resection procedure,

where the doctor slices into the bladder nodule so pieces of it can be sent to the lab for evaluation. Ten days later I got the good news – Stage 2 muscle-invasive bladder cancer. The good news out of all of this, my doctor indicated, was that usually there are no symptoms with early onset bladder cancer. I can recall sitting in the little exam room with my husband as we waited for the doctor to come in. It was quiet as all of the other patients for the day had gone — this must be the time of the day for BAD NEWS. I wasn't sure of what he was going to say. When he finally said those awful words, "bladder cancer" I was stunned. But he did indicate that symptoms don't rear their ugly heads until much later, when there may not be much hope. So, the pain in my back was a help.

Little comfort to me.

Two days later I landed in the ER again. This time the pain was beyond severe. Morphine helped and once the pain subsided, the nurses told me to stay as hydrated as possible. Thank God, the pain did not return, for some strange reason.

No one to my knowledge had ever had bladder cancer in my family. My mom suffered with rheumatoid arthritis, my dad had Type 2 diabetes. I always took after my mom physiologically and she never had any cancer of any kind; just varicose vein surgery when I was a kid. I wasn't a smoker nor did I work in places where certain chemicals polluted the air all day long.

My next stop was to the oncologist. This was getting serious. At first, treatment was to be eight weeks of two chemotherapy drugs. Then the doctor switched it out to four chemo drugs every two weeks for four infusions. Otherwise, he said, it would be too tiring for me. He couldn't have been more right. By Halloween, chemo would be finished. Haha.

At this point, I was reading everything I could about bladder cancer. The stages and life expectancies. Some articles said things I liked, others were not so nice. Five years, no you can live longer than that. Depending on if the cancer comes back, don't be too optimistic. Wait! Someone's relative had bladder cancer 16 years ago and they're still living. It scared me terribly.

For the first time in all my life, I was faced with death. An early death, as far as I was concerned. I was 66 years old, and FULL of life! There were so many things I was doing, and so many things I had yet to do – how could I think on dying. I want to see my grand daughters grow up. I want to write that mystery novel I've been planning. I want to visit Graceland. There are many more trips to places we love to visit every year, that I wanted to just keep doing!

Muscle-invasive cancer is aggressive. It grows fast. It had to be stopped. Like standing with your hand up on the tracks staring down the freight train. That's how I felt my odds were. I am in control! Only sadly, I knew I was not. Not anymore, if I ever had been.

Was I afraid to die? Yes.

And no.

It began to occur to me that God is in control. Not me. God.

Father, Son and Holy Spirit.

CHAPTER ONE

THERE IS ANTICIPATION HERE

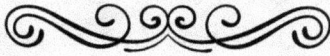

I n all my long life, I am 67 years old, never, ever did it ever occur to me that cancer would be a part of my world. I don't even have high blood pressure. Year in and year out my health just seemed to be something to be relegated to the back burner. Yes, I have seasonal allergies, and sneezing from dog fur and mold, but it is being cared for.

When the urology doctor held the pathology report in his hands and softly told me and my husband Bob that I did have bladder cancer, I was stunned. Into silence. What do you say? Stage 2, he said, which means it has invaded the muscle wall. It's aggressive, so it will have to be treated aggressively.

By the middle of August 2018, I was seeing an oncology doctor who told me it would be eight treatments every two weeks. Then just before chemotherapy started, he changed the regimen to four chemo infusions. By the end of September, I started my first chemotherapy treatment.

I was almost excited to be on this road. After all, it occurred to me on a daily basis that cancer was growing inside me and I had no idea how bad it was getting. This was an experience that I would now be living. There was anticipation here.

After the first few days following chemotherapy, nausea set in, then vomiting. I was tired but the fatigue wasn't too bad. No hair loss to speak of. Then I developed metal mouth. It is the sensation that everything tastes like gun metal. It was awful. It lasted for about five days, then was gone, never to return. By the second infusion, I broke out with mouth sores. They give you a Magic Mouthwash, which isn't bad, but didn't do much to counteract all the sores in my mouth.

Throughout my life I have lived with canker sores. Usually only one at a time, but their ferocity is such that you wouldn't want more than one. On a few occasions, I had thrush mouth from an antibiotic, which was similar to this. Because this mouthful of sores was something I had encountered before, I just lived with it until it went away. Thank goodness, it never returned.

Vinblastine. A medication to treat bladder cancer. Doxorubicin. Another medication to treat cancer. Methotrexate. An injection to treat bladder cancer. Cisplatin. The side effects for this drug can take up an entire page when you go looking for information. A few of these drugs went directly in the port and a few were done by "push", where the nurse would slowly inject the medication into the IV. The oncology nurses were fabulous. They see this every week, every month, yet they treat you with a kindness that is all yours.

The nurses would start off with sodium chloride liquid, seeping into my veins for two hours. Then would come the anti-nausea drugs, two of those. Finally, I would receive the four chemotherapy drugs, one at a time, then two more hours of sodium chloride to flush it all out. A full day. I would feel relatively alright when it was all over.

By the third infusion my white blood cell count was so low, they had to postpone the infusion for a week. Great, I thought, instead of being done by Halloween, now I would have to tack on an additional week. By this time, I was feeling beyond awful, if there is such a feeling. Fatigue had me napping two to three hours every afternoon.

Slowly my appetite went away. Drink, they say, drink lots of water! Only problem with this is that water was 'toxic' to my body. Just a little sip and I would throw it right back up. I don't know why, that's just the way it was. So, it was on to fruit juices because tea and coffee tasted terribly odd. The only comfort I found was in a daily morning chocolate Boost drink. It wasn't much, yet it stayed down.

For the rest of the day(s), I would sip juice or try broth or soup. Nothing much and some days I couldn't look at food. That day would flow into the next and then the next, and some weeks, I wasn't eating for four or five days in a row. Great way to lose weight.

By the fourth infusion, again I had it postponed a week because I was looking and feeling like death warmed over. Every time I went in for a chemotherapy infusion, I was there for about six hours every time. It was a full day of sitting in the infusion room getting drugs in and then having them flushed out. All this anticipation for chemotherapy had led me to a dead-end to my life.

The side effects were worst of all. The ever-present fatigue, nausea, vomiting every day every day, no appetite, weight loss, my hair slowly falling out, mouth sores, bone pain, dizziness, weakness beyond what you can imagine. Thick saliva which was the worst thing of all. When I mentioned it to the doctor in Philadelphia, he just nodded his head and said it is another side effect, and it will go away in time. Just a life of misery.

And then there was the nephrostomy tube. Stuck into my right kidney from my back, I lived with this thing from the day after Labor Day until the surgery on December 17. It wasn't too bad, all things considered, but by the end of October it started leaking. Not good.

So, another trip to the radiology department for them to replace the tube. It was a simple procedure, just taking one tube out of my kidney and putting another one in — but it was one of the most painful experiences of my life. I was in agony on that little table waiting for them to finish.

The doctor and nurses couldn't understand why I would have pain, but my oncologist later told me it was probably due to the fact that my body just couldn't take any more poking around at that point. It was something that shouldn't have been done, but I had no choice.

All my life I have been a busy person. Taking night classes, raising a family, working fulltime, keeping a beautiful home, cooking, baking, knitting, writing, keeping pets – these were my life! Even after my daughter and son grew up and moved away, there was still plenty to do. And now I was sitting in a recliner hour after hour, doing nothing.

And I do mean nothing.

Then there were those long drives out to Philadelphia from Ocean County, NJ. If we had a 7:30 a.m. appointment, we had to leave the house by 5 or 5:30 because you never knew what you would encounter all along the way. That endless bumpy ride on Route 70, driving in the dark, traveling along 295 South, then 76 West, and sometimes watching the moon travel with us, made my upset stomach a little more upset. By the time we would pull into the parking garage at the Perelman Center for Advanced Medicine, I would get out and spend a few minutes dry retching in front of the car.

WHY DO WE SUFFER? That is the question for the ages. Most often we will hear from someone who will inevitably say, "why does God allow suffering?" Often, that person is no longer interested in their faith; they have walked away due to some episode in their life that didn't turn out as planned. But, planned by who? Just why is it that God allows suffering?

Well, he really doesn't. He gives us Free Will. Now that doesn't mean we go ahead and "find" cancer or tumors or precarious ways of living that put us on death's precipice. There are circumstances in our lives which may cause us to feel stress beyond what we can endure, and something inside of us goes awry. Our physiology gets all messed up. Hence the cancer or the tumor or the big problem.

I never referred to my bladder cancer as "my cancer." I didn't want to own it. It was a part of my physical makeup at that point, but nothing I had invited in. So, it was as if I had an unwanted guest who had come for dinner and refused to go. Through chemo drugs and surgery, I was eventually able to push this unwarranted pest out the door. But, it took a LOT of doing.

That is why we are so lucky to experience suffering!

What!, you're thinking! Yes, suffering. Didn't the good Lord say: "give thanks in all circumstances; for this is God's will for you in Christ Jesus." 1 Thessalonians 5:18.

Well, that is of little comfort when I was enduring a daily dose of nausea and vomiting for days on end. I had not the strength to get off my recliner, not do anything at all. Not even pray. Eventually, there were hours when the sick feelings would subside and I would take up my rosary and say a decade or two. I would also say a prayer to Jesus giving him my suffering for that day.

That is called redemptive suffering. We do not suffer for no reason. And when we are faced with life's trials and tribulations, we can give them in their entirety over to the Lord. Many was the day I would tell Jesus that "here is my suffering and I am laying it at the foot of your cross. Please in your mercy, sometime this day, look down and take this suffering to yourself."

Crawl beneath the cross and lay there. Feel close to Mary and Jesus. Sometimes that is all you can do. Tell Jesus you are here, look down and see me, know that I love you more than my life. Then be still in the knowledge that the Lord knows you are there, He knows what is wrong and He will let you suffer still with Him. Remember, the salvation of the world was not achieved but through suffering!

Remember, too, that God the Father has given you a piece of his Son's cross to be with you in your affliction. Whatever that may be, and we all have struggles, trials, difficulties and sorrows in our lives, we need to think on the Cross, grab onto the splintery wood and never let go.

THAT is how we can give thanks to God in all circumstances. He is not asking us to be glad that we have cancer or a brain tumor or that a family member has been tragically killed in a car accident; what He is asking us to do is to always remember that He is with us through every occasion we find ourselves in. That our suffering is His suffering, that our suffering is Mary's suffering.

And as Fr. John Paul Mary said in his homily on the feast of Our Lady of Lourdes, "suffering is meant to bring more love."

A truth to live by.

"Weeping may last through the night, but joy comes in the morning." Psalm 30:5

The anticipation of Advent teaches us many things. We learn to look ahead, to cherish what is coming; through the lighting of the Advent candles week by week, to opening the windows of our Advent calendars, to reading the prayers and gospels on a daily basis.

Going through this Advent of 2018, also taught me that it is in the present moment that we live. The here-and-now. Truthfully, there is no other time.

All had been removed from me. I had not the strength nor the desire to walk my dogs, or even to pick up a knitting needle. Nothing appeared worth doing. I wasn't in a depressed state of mind, just so weak and powerless that to undertake anything was beyond my capacity, that day or the next week.

Those early days of Advent taught me something I had never thought of prior: all those "things" which we so highly prize in our lives, that we simply cannot live without, we can live without. They make up the busy hours of our days, and we think we cannot live without them – all those things are passing things.

We can live without them. What we cannot live without is prayer.

Advent is a holy season in the Catholic church, much like Lent, Pentecost, Easter, and Ordinary Time. These four weeks should be lived in a joyful expectation of what is to come. We are a hopeful people, even in the midst of difficulties, even as we still stand beneath the cross with Mary, and keep our Lord company.

Learn to do this through prayerful penance and preparing

spiritually for Jesus Christ. Advent is the connection between so many things, events and people. It is our gift to God.

And when we realize what has been gained by it, we see how it has always been God's gift to us. He has given us not only the traditions and devotions of this holy season, but we are in the midst of the Blessed Virgin Mary as she, with us, prepares for the coming of Jesus.

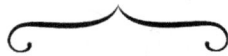

Prayer for Those in Their Last Agony

(Recited while kneeling)

O Most Merciful Jesus, Lover of Souls:

I pray Thee, by the agony of Thy most Sacred Heart,

and by the sorrows of Thine Immaculate Mother,

cleanse in Thy Blood the sinners of the whole world who are now in their last agony,

and are to die this day. Amen.

Heart of Jesus, Agonizing, have mercy on the dying.

Jesus, Mary, Joseph, we love Thee, save souls.

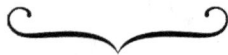

CHAPTER TWO

DECEMBER DARKNESS

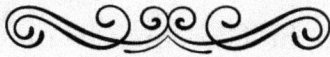

ecember gets dark early. By 5:00 p.m. it's dark out there. Many people don't like those early sunsets. I happen to like them a lot. Perhaps because I've always loved books and having it grow dark outside early, was simply another excuse to sit down and read.

By the time we roll into December, darkness has been with us for quite some time. November doesn't disappoint and when we lived in New Hampshire, many was the day when it was genuinely dark by 4:30. When we lived in Pennsylvania, the sun would set behind a hill in our wooded backyard, where suddenly all the light would be gone from our street. If you climbed to the top of that hill, you would have seen the sun still there, but it was gone from my sight.

Advent sometimes feels like that. Especially now in our culture; we are supposed to be in some kind of Christmas frenzy the minute the kids take off their Halloween costumes. After all, those shopping channels on TV are all decked out with their 'holiday' glitz. And the minute it's December 26th, well goodbye to Christmas.

But, Advent was the 28 days before Christmas Day and the season of Christmas is just beginning on Dec. 26. At times it seems to me as if the season of Advent has fallen behind that high Pennsylvania hill where no one sees it. Or, at the very least, pays much attention to it.

In order to have a 'right' Christmas you must pay attention to what precedes it. That most beautiful season of Advent. The word itself is derived from the Latin word adventus, which means "coming". Advent is a time of preparation, prayer, fasting and penance. Most often we are all caught up in shopping, baking, decorating and partying. No wonder when December 25 comes, we're left speculating on 'what just happened here'.

Advent, then, is waiting and preparing for the Christ-child, but it is also anticipating His coming again. How we approach Advent will set the tone for our Christmas celebrations and all that follow in the days after the 'big day' itself.

When I was very young, we would attend an Advent supper every year at my father's church. I say that because my father was not Catholic, he was Lutheran. On occasion my mother, sister and I would attend a function at St. Paul's. The supper was always packed jammed and we would see the same people there every year. My aunt Louise and uncle Rick would be there and Santa usually made an appearance toward the end of the night. The food was brought in by the church-goers and after eating, all the Advent wreath supplies would be handed out.

I still remember the light, the warmth and the goodness of being there. Opening the door to the ladies restroom, many times someone forgot to turn on the heat and it would be freezing cold in there. I don't believe that building is even there anymore; the church itself has gone over to another denomination, but still stands in the neighborhood.

That yearly Advent supper is one of my best childhood memories. Maybe it was all the people there, the goodwill, the conversations, the happiness of the event. It didn't matter to me that it wasn't 'Catholic', it was real and it was pointed towards God.

That's what Advent is, a signpost pointing to the coming of Jesus. There is the signpost of awareness, that we should be paying attention to what is coming; there is the signpost of John the Baptist proclaiming there is someone greater than himself that will be coming. Then, there is another signpost we Catholics trust in to point us to Jesus – His mother, Mary.

Mary is my everything.

Some Christian believers believe that Catholics such as I worship Mary. We do not. She is not part of the Trinity; she was as human as you and me. Why then, do we pay so much attention to her?

You would be a fool not to include Mary in your Catholic devotions. My mother taught me that from when I was very young. "Turn to Mary in everything" she always told me. I do that everyday, I have done that all my life, and I did that on the day my mother was laid to rest, one of the saddest days of my life.

This is why I love our Church so much. We have been given the saints. We can rely on their words and wisdom. They struggled through life just as we do. Many of them came very late to the faith; yet come they did. They were known for doing everything there was to do in life, but something or some way drew them to God, where they never departed.

Let me tell you about Mary first. Then about a most extraordinary man, Saint Maximilian Kolbe.

The Blessed Virgin Mary is always popular at Christmas. After all, she's there, in the manger, as a significant player, and you just can't ignore her. To some Christians Mary is then relegated to the shelf or closet until December rolls around once again.

There is not a day goes by that Mary is not in my life. She is, after all, the Mother of God.

Our Lady of the Rosary. Our Lady of Lourdes, of Fatima, Undoer of Knots, the Blessed Virgin, Theotokos, Star of the Sea, Rosa Mystica, Queen of Heaven, the Black Madonna of Czestochowa, Our Lady of Guadalupe, Our Lady of Perpetual Help, Morning Star, Gate of Heaven, Holy Mary, Help of the Afflicted, Queen of Martyrs, Queen of Apostles, Our Lady of Grace, the Immaculate Conception and so many other titles are all the same woman. They are all names for Mary.

As a diamond shining brightly in the darkness, Mary illuminates for us just how she figures in God's plan of salvation. Jesus, after all, gave her to not only John but to all of us, too. Our Lord told Mary to "behold her son", – and that is all of us. Speaking to Mary on Calvary, He wasn't making plans at that moment for Mary's residency concerns.

Whatever name you call Mary by, she never lets you down. That is because Mary intercedes for us. She is our go-between for getting to Jesus. And why go to Mary and not Jesus directly?

If you've ever been told that Catholics worship Mary like God, you've been told something WRONG! Catholics believe that worship is only God's alone. We believe in the Holy Trinity, Father, Son and Holy Spirit. There is no other "god" that stands in for our one and triune God. There is Jesus Christ, true God and true man, and our only hope of salvation.

So, why go to Mary first?

"The Blessed Mother comes instantly to your side to pray with you. And she does not come alone.

She brings angels with her. And not just one or two for she is the Queen of angels, so choirs of angels come with her. And she and Jesus are joined at the heart and cannot be separated so she brings Jesus with her.

And Jesus cannot be separated from The Trinity so He brings The Father and The Holy Spirit with Him. And where The Holy Trinity is all creation is...

Is it any wonder that anyone who prays the rosary from the heart is so blessed and protected and powerful in their prayers for others?" -Fr. Amorth, Chief Exorcist for the Vatican

We venerate Mary. We do not worship her as a god. Anyone who tells you that doesn't know what they're talking about. We honor our Blessed Mother as the Mother of God and we turn to her as we do to all the rest of the Communion of Saints that we have to call on in our rich Catholic heritage. Mary is God's perfect love. Even though she was born, just like all of us, she was preserved from sin, the original sin, that everyone else has initially.

God did this in order that Mary would be ready to bring forth her Son in due time. Nothing else would do. Her role is one that constantly points to Jesus. She is, as St. Louis de Montfort points out, the echo of God. Whatever God says, Mary echoes. She doesn't make any of it up herself.

Mary only exalts her Son. Her role as Mother of God or Theotokos, is meant to glorify Jesus Christ and in its own way to honor Mary. Her beautiful prayer known as the Magnificat, gives all glory to God, not to herself. In his perfect way, God sees to it that Mary's role in the Church is one of courage; her trust in God totally brings our faith and love to perfection, as it was meant to do.

Mary does not say to us, "pray to me and I will give you miracles." Rather, she say, "pray to me and I will grant you graces; graces for your life and I will turn to my Son with your needs."

Mary's humility, her hidden way, her whole life is simply to be emulated by faithful Catholics and that is why we should turn to her always and learn from her. The Catechism of the Catholic Church says it this way: "Mary's role in the Church is inseparable from her union with Christ and flows directly from it". (CCC 964)

The Blessed Virgin is our Mediatrix and Co-Redemptrix. Just as every day when going through chemotherapy I was barely able to function in any kind of right way, Mary was there for me as she is for every weary traveler along the way. She is a welcome respite, one who hears our petitions, comforts us and never, ever lets us down. She turns to her Son and gives him our news. There is no one like her.

Catholic teaching as regards Mary means that Our Lady protects and guards mightily God's plan of salvation for all of us. Our suffering, whatever it is, is redemptive; that is, we can give it to Jesus through Mary, as a way of uniting our pains to His cross. Suffering is not in vain. It may be awful, it may be unbearable, but there is a comfort that in our suffering we are united with Jesus on the cross. That suffering, our suffering, is used by God in a way that is unknown to us to bring comfort and relief to others. There are just some things in this life that will forever remain a mystery until the next life.

In our Catholic faith, we are blessed to have four Marian dogmas. These are principles of our faith that the Church has said are true and we should believe in them. Marian dogmas are:

Mary, Mother of God

Perpetual Virginity

The Immaculate Conception

The Assumption

I'm hoping and praying that in the near future a fifth Marian dogma will be announced, one entitled Co-Redemptrix, Mediatrix of All Graces, Advocate.

We are, after all, living in the Age of Mary. This is why a Fifth Marian Dogma is so necessary. For genuine love of Mary can only begin with genuine knowledge about who Mary is. She lived, acted, thought and suffered in the exact ways Our Lord did. There was nothing He experienced that she did not; and that included the crucifixion. Her own heart was pierced.

It was through Mary's sufferings too, that she took part in the redemption of the world. She truly is co-redemptrix.

All graces, all favors come from Mary. She is known as the Mediatrix of all graces. It is through the intercession of Mary that we enjoy the graces set upon this world through the redemption of Jesus Christ. This motherly intercession started with Mary's "yes" at the Annunciation, when Mary agreed, fearful as she was, to become the Mother of God. That is what she is to each one of us, and we recite that every time we say a 'Hail Mary'.

Lastly, Mary is our first intercessor after Jesus. She takes any and all of our petitions that we lay before her, to her Son. She asks of Him as she did at the wedding feast of Cana, where Christ's earthly miracles would commence. Especially in times of trials, difficulties, sickness, darkness, and despair, Our Lady never leaves our side. Best of all, she brings her Son to help us fully.

Salvation is through Jesus Christ alone. But, and don't ever underestimate a "but" from God, this work of salvation is to be accomplished with the help of a woman. Specifically our Blessed Mother. Remember, this first appeared in Genesis 3:15 – "I will put enmity between you and the woman, and between your seed and her seed: she shall crush your head."

This is a struggle, this is an ongoing battle that will, ultimately, be won by us with our Lady's help. This is why we turn to Mary with our every petition, this is why Mary is so vitally important to us. Her 'collaboration' with her Son is recognized in the Church as "Marian co-redemption". It never precedes the Lord or eclipses him. It remains secondary and takes nothing away from the glory of our Lord.

But, here's the thing. God has given each of us a portion of His glory to take into the world. He did this for Mary, too. It was her "yes" to God that brought forth Jesus into our world. She became the Co-Redemptrix the very minute she gave her assent.

Mary's entire life was lived in Jesus. It was sharing in His redemptive mission to the world. There are numerous examples of how this played out, such as her meeting with Simeon in the temple, the wedding feast at Cana and especially her standing beneath the cross as her son was dying.

Mary gave Jesus his human nature. She said yes and in so doing, she became the "bearer of God". She is a go-between for us and Jesus. She is a mediator. At Calvary didn't Jesus give us his mother? He made Mary the Mother of All Christians and she is here to take our prayers to Him whenever we call on her.

By Mary's intercession for us, she becomes our Advocate. When we say "Mary", she says "Jesus". Nothing is her own, she gives our petitions and prayers to Jesus Christ. Mary is our Co-Redemptrix, our Mediatrix and our Advocate. THIS is why we pray to Mary. THIS is why the Blessed Virgin is of vital importance to all of us.

From my earliest memories, I can recall my mother always telling me to turn to Mary with all of my worries and concerns. A day does not go by that I am not saying a rosary to give to our blessed Lord. Her graces and love cannot be surpassed by anyone, save by our Lord.

Even when I felt so sick that I couldn't pray, I would still make the sign of the cross and ask Mary to just be with me that day.

To this day, I know she was there.

Be one with Mary. Make her a part of your life. Learn Marian devotions, get her prayer books, find out for yourself what she means to us and to the Church. And remember this:

The road with Mary will be narrow, it will be rocky, it will be difficult and you will suffer. You won't find a lot of other people there. But the ones you do meet will be with you for the journey.

And your eyes will be opened like never before. Advent can take you to our Lady. Be ready for her. In those dark evenings of

December, be quiet, and be little. Stay hidden in Our Lady.

"Let those who think that the Church pays too much attention to Mary give heed to the fact that Our Blessed Lord Himself gave ten times as much of His life to her as He gave to His Apostles."

Venerable Archbishop Fulton J. Sheen

The World's First Love: Mary, Mother of God

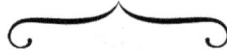

MEMORARE

Remember, O most gracious Virgin Mary,

that never was it known that anyone who fled to thy
protection,

implored thy help, or sought thine intercession was left
unaided.

Inspired by this confidence, I fly unto thee,

O Virgin of virgins, my mother;

to thee do I come, before thee I stand,

sinful and sorrowful.

O Mother of the Word Incarnate,

despise not my petitions,

but in thy mercy hear and answer me. Amen.

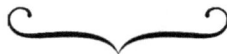

CHAPTER THREE

LIVE THE VIRTUES

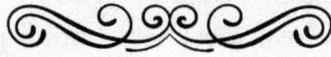

A virtue, according to the Catholic Church, is a good habit which enables people to act according to right reason enlightened by their faith. Virtues are like a good habit; something we should be practicing all our lives. Virtues go way beyond feeling like a goody-two-shoes. We are to seek out the goodness in the world; and only by living our lives in virtuous ways will those virtues become stronger. Or weaker, if we choose to walk away from them.

It's a hard thing indeed to care about virtues when you are staring down nausea every day. I never strayed far from the bathroom, for good reason, and any time I had to visit the doctor's office, I was sure to take a large plastic bowl with me in the car. (That bowl has since been thrown away.)

Anti-nausea pills didn't do much for me. There were some pills that came back up the minute they were swallowed. Eating was almost non-existent. There would be a string of days where nothing was consumed save for a Boost chocolate drink and some juice sipped all day long. It sure helped to get those extra pounds shed, but, I wouldn't recommend this diet to anyone.

Virtues, from a Catholic perspective, define who we are and how we live. There are the Cardinal virtues of prudence, justice, fortitude and temperance. There are the Theological virtues of Faith, Hope and Charity. There are the Capital virtues of chastity, generosity, temperance, brotherly love, meekness, humility and diligence.

I would also include in this list the virtue of surrender. Living with cancer and fighting it aggressively doesn't mean you surrender; no, what it denotes is that you give your life over to the Lord. You can do that in any number of ways, through direct prayer to God, through a saint's intercession, through asking family and friends to pray for you, or through asking Our Lady to turn to Jesus on your behalf.

I did all of these things. There was no knowing how things were progressing inside of me. Was the cancer being stopped through chemo or was it still expanding or had it reached other places? That last, was my biggest fear. Yet, sitting in my recliner, made me realize I had no control over any of it. Even once the chemo was finished and the surgery was scheduled, there was nothing I could do. Only surrender it all to God.

From just sitting quietly, doing 'nothing' all day long, gave me lots of time to think. I understood that humility is not a quitting or keeping my head down directive. Humility simply means my life is 100% in the hands of God. Everything there is has come from Him. To believe that we are in control is a sentiment best left to high school days.

Some virtues sound so weak, don't they? Humility is one, meekness is another. Just what does God intend for those he has put on earth? That we run and hide or stop in fear whenever trouble overtakes us? Well no, those are the times when we can turn to the Theological virtues of faith, hope and charity.

Look up Hebrews 11:1. "Now faith is the assurance of things hoped for, the conviction of things not seen." If we have a solid Catholic upbringing, we recognize that faith is not only a virtue, but an intellectual virtue. This faith plays itself out in our daily lives, in everything we do and say and think. All of our actions are based on what we believe in our hearts.

The virtue of hope keeps us going. We all have happy times and sad times. Even dry times, when prayer does not seem to matter much or we fill up our days with so much else, there's no time for prayer. Those times when we are mocked, face adversity or betrayal and for all those dry times, our hope lies in Jesus Christ. It really was the only thing left to me as I struggled to get through each day.

Charity taught me so many things. It is my love for family, friends, and neighbors. In a time when I couldn't reach out in any way to anyone, they reached out to me instead. Family members that I hadn't heard from in quite some time, would call or send encouragement to me. Even Facebook postings meant so much to me. Never believe your reaching out to others in times of trouble is a waste of time. Gestures such as these are always welcome. Charity as a virtue means through all these people, my love for God grows more steady and more tantamount in my life. Nothing is above my God.

One other virtue I learned to love was patience. Feeling sick on a daily basis is no fun. Some people liken chemotherapy to a bad case of the flu; I would say it goes way beyond that. Depending on what drugs you are given, you might not feel too bad at all. My oncologist told me that in order to fight an aggressive cancer such as stage two muscle-invasive bladder cancer, you have to fight it aggressively. That's what he did.

Day by day it was hard living. The only respite I got was to lay down and close my eyes to it all. There was nothing else I could do. I felt so sick. And tired. And weak. And good for nothing.

Patiently I waited for things to get better. It didn't happen for many weeks. So, I came to understand that being patient is also a virtue to be learned well. This was my season of cancer. It was only a season and like any season, it will pass away.

Hour after hour would go by and I was still sitting there. Thoughts would come and go in my head, and where I would at any other time get up and make a note of something remarkable, now I just sat there and let thoughts float away. But, it was okay, it was meant to be this way. Days of nothing.

Or you could say, 'appearances are deceiving'. In those so-called empty days, I learned a most valuable lesson: that my life is truly in God's hands. Whatever happens, happens. This was the time for me to do nothing. No dog-walking, no knitting, no reading, no cleaning, no cooking, no dishwashing, no vacuuming, no driving, no babysitting, no TV watching, no food shopping, no online shopping, no email checking, no traveling, no visiting, no writing, no laundry, no doing of any kind.

All these things had been taken away from me. But, only for a while. They would return, as they have now, in the writing of this book. Most of my energy is back and the chemo fatigue is gone, thank the Lord.

As you can see, virtues are a most beautiful thing. They are the WAY we should all be striving to live our lives; in good ways without much diversion or guilt over still not getting it right. Getting it right is a lifelong endeavor, one that will never be finished no matter how long or how short our lives turn out to be.

Virtues are how we learn to serve God entirely. It is, as Saint John Henry Newman once said, that the closer we strive to serve God, we begin to see the 'beauty of holiness' in our everyday lives. Because God is always with us; walking right beside us or sitting on the recliner with you. And me. We never walk through life alone.

The virtues, if practiced rightly, give us grace. That is their intent. As Newman observed, we are in this world to experience not just the easy and the pretty, but the toils and the troubles which seem to be around every corner.

True devotion to Mary happens when we have the deepest of love for her. She is, after all, the Mother of God. We should be imitating her virtues each and every day; those virtues of faith, chastity and charity. The modern world is in desperate need of these three virtues.

God gave me many hours of quiet. Sitting in the corner of my family room, in my recliner, there was really nothing else I could do. In these quiet times, in early December, is when the realizations came to me of all I had been given in this cancer. While things of this world had been taken away, they had been replaced by thoughts and prayers I had never imagined in all my sixty-seven years.

Life is a struggle. It is full of difficulty. I have no way of knowing if cancer will return to me again. Neither do I have any guarantee of waking up tomorrow morning or of returning home once I leave my house in the SUV. None of us knows what the future brings. We are not in control, only we fool ourselves into thinking we have all the answers and tomorrow will come, no matter what.

It is so important to understand all that we have been given. Suffering is a part of life; some people endure things a lot more than others, and I have no answer for why that is, any more than you do. That is what makes all the good times so sweet. Those delightful-filled hours overflow with gratitude once we understand who has been with us through it all.

Those months in 2018 will never be forgotten. At my lowest as a human being, I learned some of the highest virtues a mind can dwell upon. I thank God Almighty for giving me this illness. "Give thanks in all circumstances; for this is the will of God in

Christ Jesus for you." (1 Thessalonians 5:18)

I don't know how one is to praise the Lord in tragic circumstances. Where loved ones have been taken away suddenly, through illness, fire, accident, a drug overdose or some other way. I have come to realize it's not the circumstance that God wants us to rejoice in, but the opening up of new paths which are revealed to us, that we are to see. That up until now our vision has been clouded over with only the things of this world.

My eyes are open Lord, only let me see good things for you.

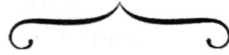

Fatima Prayer

O my Jesus,

forgive us our sins;

save us from the fires of hell.

Lead all souls to heaven,

especially those who are in most need of Your mercy.

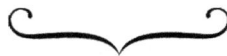

CHAPTER FOUR

I HAVE EVERYTHING

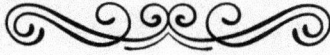

In those quiet hours when day after day I was feeling too sick to do anything, I would think about things that had come and gone in my life. It really has been a full life. Filled to the brim with family, good times, not-so-good times, places, vistas, seasons and everything that a life should be. I have been blessed to be married to a good man and have two grown children and grandchildren. My dogs are my kids, too. They depend on us for everything.

Funny how that word keeps popping up. Listening to classical music as it rolled out of my radio all day long, my mind would wander back to when my husband and I were innkeepers in New Hampshire. I simply loved that 1853 Greek Revival bed and breakfast we called home. We had 10 guest rooms and usually during the winter months we didn't have many guests on weekdays.

That gave me the opportunity to visit each guest room; straightening bed linens, checking on supplies, polishing furniture, making sure the candles in the windows were straight and secure. Once it grew dark, that was a special time for wandering. I would sit on one of the two single beds in that first floor guest room, sit near the windows and feel the heat of the radiator in front of me. I would watch cars driving by and see the snow softly falling. It was a moment in time I will always remember.

Walking the upstairs hallway, I would catch a glimpse of that lone candle sconce on the wall right outside one of the guest rooms further down the hall. If you glanced down the long back hall, you could see that electric candle softly lighting the way into the guest room there. The third floor guest room offered front and back views of the outdoor surroundings and the sun would pour forth up there like maple syrup on pancakes. It was so beautiful!

It was a struggle staying in New Hampshire and we were gone from there in three years. But, I must say my life has been very blessed. Along the way I guess you could say I had everything.

A nice upbringing, married young, had my children, Stephanie and Rob, by the time I was 25, owned homes, found jobs, went back to school for a four-year degree, owned pets, had the ability to have new cars and new clothes, had lots of family to fall back on, and even had those family members who turned out to be not so nice.

Everything.

Since my cancer diagnosis, being at Mass every week is vitally important to me. It defines who I am. Even with all of the scandals and upsets going on in the Church these days, I can still pray every day that everything I've been given stays on track, and Lord give me the strength to deal with things, if they ever do go astray.

Prayers are one of the things we have so much of in our Catholic faith. If you don't have a good Catholic prayer book, by all means get yourself one. I have recommendations at the end of this book, for all of the books that mean so much to me, so take a look there.

Advent is a time to renew our prayer time anyway. There are the Liturgy of the Hours, the Magnificat, (a monthly publication which I highly recommend), the Rosary, and all of our prayers which can be found just about anywhere. There are Catholic apps, such as EWTN, iBreviary, Discerning Hearts, Laudate, The Holy Rosary and dozens more. You can even find apps to help you make a good confession.

The Advent liturgy emphasizes awaiting Jesus but also keeps Mary front and center for us. This beautiful, prayerful season is a time of quiet devotion to the Mother of God. I think she would like it that way.

Didn't Jesus say "when you pray, go into your room and shut the door and pray to your Father who is in secret and your Father who sees in secret will reward you. (Matthew 6:6) Mary has been this way all her life. It is just her way and so opposite to what modern life is like. Be like Mary; if only for 30 minutes each day.

Within Advent itself, are beautiful Marian feast days, beginning with the Solemnity of the Immaculate Conception on December 8th. Many people, even Catholics, may tell you that this holy day means Jesus was conceived without sin, which is wrong. Mary was conceived without original sin because there needed to be a pure and sinless conception for anyone who would eventually be the mother of our Lord.

There is also the feast of Our Lady of Loreto on December 10th and the celebration of Our Lady of Guadalupe on December 12th. So many ways to honor our Mother. It is so because Mary wants to help us prepare our hearts for bringing forth Christ for her at Christmas.

Mary gives us abundant graces. If you don't feel particularly blessed lately, talk to Mary like a mother and ask her for graces. You won't be disappointed.

You know, having 'everything' does not make us happy. No matter how much stuff you or I can fill our lives with, those material things will never quite fulfill us. There will always be a part of us that does not feel entirely sated. This is God's way. And if we're intuitive enough, we will turn to Him for ways to be made whole while living on this earth.

As Catholics, we are so blessed to have the blessings of the saints who have gone before us. They are like a light on our paths, as we read and learn more about who they were, the things they did, the ways in which they suffered and how they led their lives.

We are all called to be saints, too. I have my favorites, such as St.

Therese of Lisieux, St. Francis de Sales, St. Louis de Montfort, and St. Peter. There is one in particular who has captured my heart; St. Maximilian Kolbe.

I don't know how many churches in the USA are named for this wonderful man, but there is a church in Toms River, New Jersey that carries his name. Maximilian Kolbe may be a contemporary saint for our day, but if you asked him, he would have told you he was nothing more than a Catholic priest.

That is what he replied when the SS guards at Auschwitz asked him who he was, when he offered to take the place of another man who was chosen to go into the starvation bunker to die. This man cried out that he had a wife and children, and Maximilian Kolbe offered to take his place.

Father Kolbe started out life in Poland which in 1894 was still a part of the Russian Empire. When he was 12 years old, he had a vision of the Blessed Virgin Mary. This would strongly influence the rest of his life. As a young teen, Maximilian and his elder brother joined the Conventual Franciscans. This was where he was given his religious name of Maximilian.

In 1917, Maximilian Kolbe organized the Militia Immaculatae to pray for the conversion of sinners and enemies against the Catholic Church, in particular the Freemasons. The following year, 1918, he was ordained a priest. All his life, Fr. Kolbe worked tirelessly promoting Mary all throughout his native Poland. He even founded a monthly publication, called Knights of the Immaculate. He traveled to India and Japan and started monasteries there.

By 1936 his poor health forced him to return to Poland once again. When the Nazis invaded his town he was arrested and jailed for three months, then released. But, trouble was never far behind him. In February 1941 the monastery where he was living was shut down. Fr. Kolbe was arrested again and taken to the Pawiak prison. By late Spring he was transferred to Auschwitz.

Fr. Kolbe maintained a calm persona throughout his incarceration in the death camp. He treated everyone the same, fellow prisoners and Nazi guards. Often a guard would shout at him to "stop looking at me" as if Fr. Kolbe could see inside his soul.

Once he had offered up his life in exchange for the other prisoner, he spent two weeks in the starvation bunker and prayed and led the prisoners in hymns and songs as they slowly starved to death. He was the last of the prisoners to be alive when the Nazi guards opened the bunker. They killed him with an injection of carbolic acid.

All his life, Fr. Kolbe had always said that his wish was for his ashes to somehow be scattered over the earth in reverence to Mary. He died on the eve of the feast of the Assumption, August 14 and the very next day he was cremated. It was then that his ashes scattered into the wind on the Feast of the Assumption.

Coincidence? I hardly think so.

Is there any more beautiful name for our Blessed Mother than the Immaculata?!

Doesn't this name just say it all. This is the name that Maximilian

Kolbe called Our Lady. This was the name that he thought about her with all the time. His entire life was given over to Mary, in everything he did, in everything he said, in the way that he lived everyday.

Maximilian Kolbe thought about our Blessed Mother all the time. He believed that there was the closest of relationship between Mary and the Holy Spirit. Fr. Kolbe wanted all peoples to come to know Our Lady. He consecrated himself to her every day and wants for us to do the same.

Fr. Kolbe believed you turn over your life to Mary. You literally put your life in her hands. As St. John Paul II's motto reminds us "Totus Tuus" – "Totally Yours". We become an instrument of Mary, we can be molded and shaped by her to do the work of God.

We are to be real Militants for the Lord and that is why Fr. Kolbe created the Knights of the Immaculate.

"We have to win the universe and each individual soul, now and in the future, down to the end of time, for the Immaculata, and by her for the Sacred Heart of Jesus. Further, we must be on the watch so that nobody tears any soul away from its consecration to the Immaculata; we should strive rather that souls may constantly deepen their love for her; that the bond of love between her and these souls may grow ever closer, and that these souls may henceforth be one with her, with her alone. This is how the Immaculata is able to live and love and act in these souls and through them. (Immaculate Conception and the Holy Spirit, pg. 114-115)

Fr. Kolbe was always taken by the name Mary proclaimed to Bernadette Soubirous, when she asked who she was speaking with, during her visions at Lourdes. "I am the Immaculate Conception" was all Mary said. Think of it this way: "Mary is Immaculate because she is the Mother of God, and she became the Mother of God because she is Immaculate." (Immaculate Conception and the Holy Spirit, pg. 151)

All my life, that phrase "Immaculate Conception" has intrigued me. It almost sounds like the least likely title Mary could have given to that young peasant girl in France, who asked the lady repeatedly who she was. And then to hear the worlds 'immaculate conception' probably made little to no sense whatsoever. One is left wondering, "huh?", what is this. Bernadette must have been wondering why those words, as they seemed to mean nothing to her. Yet these words, Immaculate Conception, were and are, the very essence of who Mary is in our world.

If you are still wondering if you should be praying to Mary, consider how St. Maximilian Kolbe wrote about it in 1938:

"From all that has been presented here we can rightly conclude that Mary as the Mother of the Savior Jesus has been made the Co-Redemptrix of the human race, and that as the Spouse of the Holy Spirit she participates in the distribution of all the graces.. ... In recent times especially we are perceiving the Immaculata, the Spouse of the Holy Spirit, as our Mediatrix." (Immaculate Conception and the Holy Spirit, pg. 169.)

If you are looking for Mary, Fr. Kolbe wrote in 1939:

"Every action has the reaction in view. The reaction is the fruit of the action. God the Father is the Primary Principle and the Last End. The Immaculata is full of grace; nothing in the way of grace is lacking to her. The path of grace is always the same: action: from the Father through the Son (Christ said, "I will send him to you"), and by the Holy Spirit (the Immaculata); then the inverse reaction: from creatures through the Immaculata (the Holy Spirit), and Christ (the Word) back to the Father. Action and reaction=love=grace and good works. (Notes, 1939) (Immaculate Conception and the Holy Spirit, pg. 39.)

Who thinks thoughts like these? Only someone covered in the mantle of Mary. Only someone who has been won over to Mary's Immaculate Heart. St. Maximilian Kolbe devoted his life to being like Mary. There is no doubt in my mind that he sits near to her for all eternity.

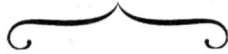

Daily Renewal of Total Consecration

Immaculata, Queen and Mother of the Church, I renew my consecration to you this day and for always, so that you may use me for the coming of the Kingdom of Jesus in the whole world. To this end I offer you all my prayers, actions and sacrifices of this day.

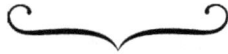

CHAPTER FIVE

I FEEL NOTHING

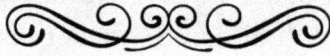

D o you sometimes feel as if you are good for nothing? Like life has passed you by, all the dreams you envisioned for yourself never having worked out? Does it seem as if you were born under an unlucky star, destined to be of little use in the whole wide world?

Don't despair. Most everyone struggles with life. Those who seem to have everything, oftentimes either don't appreciate what they have or act like they deserved it.

We are given incredible opportunities to become one of God's most useful tools. All you have to do is to recognize that your life is nothing without God and through prayer act in ways that are right for you. You'll know what they are; your 'little voice' inside your head, will keep you where you need to be.

Our culture today acts as if faith, religion, is nothing. Who needs that waste of time, anyway, some will tell you? Many who are 'famous' in movies, TV, celebrity of some kind, at their job or business, or politics seem to be as far removed from faith as you can possibly get.

I often wonder what Christmas or Advent means to a person who storms through the big box front door on Black Friday and rips merchandise away from others who are there with the same idea? Where is their sense of magnanimity, their generosity or goodwill for others? What could Advent or Christmas possibly mean to those who have no correct definition of the moment?

Years ago I worked in a local nursing home as a nursing aide. One afternoon as I was at the A-wing nurses station, one of the girls from the kitchen came over to ask for a few aspirin for a headache she had. She then proceeded to tell everyone who was there that her family wouldn't be celebrating Christmas that year.

One of the nurses asked her why. She said her father had just lost his job so there would be no money for gifts. I looked at her and said "so why can't you celebrate Christmas?"

Well, she stared back at me as if I had three heads on my shoulder and repeated that her father had lost his job. And I said to her, "what does that have to do with celebrating Christmas?" Without waiting for an answer I told her, that even if I didn't have one gift, I could still celebrate Christmas.

She said nothing, probably just thought what an idiot she was talking to. Is it not true that we can celebrate Christmas without gifts? If we can't afford them for some reason or had an emergency which precluded decorating, baking, and all the rest; couldn't we still celebrate Christmas?

Christmas is all about the gift we make of ourselves – the gift we can become for Jesus. We do that by preparing for Our Lord all during Advent. We can be the gift when there are no others. Even when it seems we have nothing to give. Even when we suffer.

When I was in the middle of chemotherapy it felt like I was on death's door. Twice my infusion date had to be pushed back because my white blood cell count was so low the oncology team didn't want to risk having me feel sicker than I already felt. It could result in fevers or hospitalization. And so another week would be stretched out in front of me; a week where nothing was accomplished.

Everything I loved doing had ground to a halt. I was living in front of a giant stop sign and could go no further. I had no desire to do anything; even when I would get dressed in the morning and attempt to make the bed, I felt so weak all I could do was sit back down again. And wait.

For what, I don't know. As the days and weeks went by it started to occur to me how most of what we fill our days with are so much frill and feathers. Most of it is so non-essential. Of course your family and your job are important but even there, things could be trimmed or done differently.

Scrolling through Facebook. Who needs it. Checking email. Another waste. Watching TV. Probably reruns. Taking another selfie. Really? Texting ad nauseum. I know the feeling only too well! Watching video's on your tablet. Leave that to the six-year-olds. Playing games on your xBox. Nothing new there. There are those, too, who do even more destructive things – like take illegal drugs or play online gambling with the mortgage money or regularly shoplift.

So many ways to waste a day. So many hours that could be used in more useful ways. I won't tell you what those are, I'm not looking to preach my way to you. What I am hoping you will see is that life only comes around once, so make the most of it.

I had nothing that once was everything and I realized that all of it was no longer needed to get through a day. I had a chair, something to drink, a radio to listen to, a window to look out of and my bed. I couldn't even appreciate my dogs and they walked around looking stressed as if they could smell the cancer (which they probably could).

I realize now that all these so-called "failures" in life are mere stepping stones that the Lord has placed in our path. These have brought us along to the place we now find ourselves in today. Whatever that place may be, we have the Lord and his Mother to guide us.

All of my desires had been changed. In a way, just like Our Lady wants us to be transformed in her. Mary wishes for each one of us to stop living for ourselves and to put our lives in her hands. She will see to it that we are pointed in the direction she has prepared for us, with the help of our Blessed Lord.

In a little book entitled "Aim Higher!", Spiritual and Marian Reflections of St. Maximilian Kolbe, this saint calls us to a life with Mary. He says, 'you will draw more knowledge about her and will be more inflamed with her love directly from her heart than from all human words put together.' (pg. 5)

Father Kolbe explains that Mary is the Mediatrix of All Graces and that the Holy Spirit does not act except through her. That is why she has been proclaimed Mediatrix. "The Immaculata is the ladder upon which we climb to the Sacred Heart of Jesus." (pg. 17) We are to strive to live a life like Jesus through Mary.

Sounds simple enough, and it can be made more so when we read the Advent scriptures daily. They help us to bring our waiting into perspective; they fill us with more and more. So we never feel as if we are nothing or have nothing.

I have everything. As Fr. Kolbe asked us to be, we should hand ourselves over to Mary, especially all of our difficulties, and for everything else, we should be at peace. "It is our ideal to win the whole world for the Immaculata and through her hands the souls who are and who will be, all of them collectively and each of them individually." (pg. 22)

Whenever I think back to those days filled with nothing I know they were that way due to the will of God. Too often we want to discern things that come our way; this cancer was not for discernment sake. It was to be embraced as something else coming to me in this life. Mary, too, suffered.

The Blessed Virgin Mary took the place of the nothingness that consumed my days in the Autumn of 2018. She became my everything. Why is that?

Did you know, Jesus saved the best for last? Dying on the cross, having been betrayed, ridiculed, stripped, scourged, spit on, made to carry his cross, crucified with nails through his hands and feet and a crown of thorns upon his head, hanging for almost three tortuous hours until He could not stay another minute, Jesus turned to His mother and said, "Woman, behold thy son. After that, he said to the disciple: Behold your mother. And from that hour the disciple took her to his own." (John 19, 25-27)

Jesus gave us his mother. He was giving Mary to all of us, IF we will have her.

She who was at first fearful then joyful at the news of the Annunciation, she who listened as Simeon pronounced that a sword would pierce her heart too, she who worried so through all the years of Jesus' growing up, she who endured scorn from so many (Who is this, Jesus, son of Mary?), she who began his ministry with a simple inquiry as to wine, she who followed and stood beneath the cross while nearly everyone else had run away. This Mary, my mother, He gave to us!

Just when it seemed all hope was gone. The disciples had fled, probably hiding away in fear for their lives, and the gift of the Holy Spirit would be given at a later date once Jesus was resurrected. At that moment, there was little to no hope. And when we're out of hope, out of everything, down to nothing, who do we call upon?

"We as Catholics need to always take Mary with us. From the Gospel of Matthew: "Do not be afraid to take Mary your wife into your home. For it is through the Holy Spirit that this child has been conceived in her." Mt. 1:20.

It is the invitation of the angel to Joseph, while he had decided to divorce her quietly. This motherhood comes from the Spirit, it is a gift of the Spirit. This is true of Mary's motherhood of Jesus and of her spiritual motherhood of us.

"She will bear a son . . . ," said the angel to Joseph.

That is what the spiritual motherhood of Mary is: to give birth to Jesus within us.

This is the motherhood of Mary: to form Jesus in us."

(Taken from the Itinerary of Preparation For Consecration to the Immaculata in The Spirit of St. Maximilian Kolbe – part 1)

There is only one name that will lead us to our Lord. One person, born of flesh just like us. One woman who will come with her Son when He returns again. Their two hearts will reign supreme. This is Mary, Mother of God.

Is there any greater gift this side of heaven?

Is there nothing in this? Or is there everything!

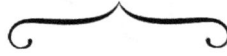

DAILY MIRACULOUS MEDAL PRAYER OF ST. MAXIMILIAN

O Mary, conceived without sin,
pray for us who have recourse to you,

and for all those who do not have recourse to you,

especially the enemies of Holy Church
and all those recommended to you.

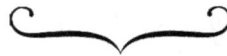

CHAPTER SIX

THE TRINITY

AND THE BLESSED VIRGIN

~~~~~~~~~~~

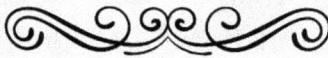

My Catholic faith revolves around two premises: the Trinity and the Eucharist. We believe in one God, but that God is Father, Son and Holy Spirit. Without the saving grace given to us on Holy Thursday by Jesus as he broke the bread and gave it to his disciples, saying "do this in memory of me" we have little to nothing to pin our hopes on in this world.

The Trinity is not of this world. Even during Advent as we wait for the coming of our Lord, we focus our attentions always on the Father, Son and Holy Spirit. I remember when I went to catechism classes and one of the sisters told us that the Trinity is a mystery; there is no way to fully understand it and we shouldn't try. We should just believe. She was right.

The Catechism of the Catholic Church puts it this way:

"The mystery of the Most Holy Trinity is the central mystery of Christian faith and life. It is the mystery of God in himself. It is therefore the source of the other mysteries of faith, the light that enlightens them. It is the most fundamental and essential teaching in the 'hierarchy of the truths of faith.' The whole history of salvation is identical with the history of the way and the means by which the one true God, Father, Son and Holy Spirit, reveals himself to men and reconciles and unites with himself those who turn away from sin." (234)

How many times during Mass do we hear the words, "through our Lord Jesus Christ, your Son, who lives and reigns with you in the unity of the Holy Spirit, one God, for ever and ever". There is your Trinity.

God the Father is God. The second Person of the Trinity, Jesus, is God. The third Person of the Trinity, the Holy Spirit is God. There are three Persons in One God. There are not three Gods. They are of the same nature, substance and being. This is not something made up by the Church; it was revealed to us by Jesus Himself. The gospel of Matthew (28:19) says, "Go teach all nations, baptizing them in the name of the Father, the Son, and the Holy Spirit."

God the Father has existed for all time. There is no beginning and no end. We can't wrap our heads around this concept, because in this world we see only 'on the surface', if you will. The Son is begotten; He comes from the Father. The Holy Spirit comes from both the Father and the Son. Each 'Person' has something to teach us about our faith; we worship and adore only God in the Trinity.

The doctrine of the Holy Trinity is the foundation of the Catholic faith; it is what everything else rests upon. The Trinity has been revealed to us, yet it truly cannot be understood by us. Oftentimes, we tend to gravitate to one or the other of the Divine Persons; and there is nothing wrong with that. Everyone has an affinity to either God the Father, God the Son or God the Holy Spirit.

During the holy season of Advent we draw near to Jesus Christ who is the One we are awaiting. At first we are told to be on the watch because the time is drawing near, then we hear from John the Baptist, and by the third Sunday of Advent, known as Gaudete Sunday, we know the time is drawing near for Our Lord to be with us. Mary, of course, figures into all of these weeks as the one who is pivotal to our understanding of the season.

We often hear the word 'conversion'. Often we think it only applies to our faith life. Yet, all of us have been on a conversion kick since we were born. We started out as babies, helpless, and in need of everything as we grew into young teens then young adults and into our middle and later years.

I recall for many years now how I love vanilla ice cream. It doesn't matter who makes it, hard or soft, whipped and swirled like what you get on the boardwalk in summer on a steaming hot day, it has been my favorite flavor. Then I went through chemotherapy. At first, I had no taste for anything, because I had no appetite for days and weeks on end.

Once I had been through the surgery, a radical cystectomy, my appetite slowly started to come around. Not everything at once mind you, things like cake, cookies and donuts had such a funny taste. Then I actually bought myself a tub of vanilla ice cream. I dished it out into a bowl and sat down to enjoy it.

It tasted awful. How could that be. I even tried it again, but couldn't eat it. So I made the switch to chocolate and that seems to satisfy. For now. There is still hope that I will get my taste back for vanilla ice cream.

Isn't conversion like that? Yes, conversion in the true Catholic sense, refers to a moral change, wherein we turn back to God and take our faith seriously. Yet, in life, often we are "dished out" events that may stop us from truly investigating our faith as we should. Especially the older we get. We "settle" for things, and then realize they are not the things we really want. It takes courage to stand apart, to stand your ground, to not follow the crowd.

It is very important to let your faith grow. If you still think the way you did when you were ten years old, it does no good to be a person of faith, for there is no faith in that. For myself, conversion has come through the reading of good Catholic books which have given me a deeper insight into what my Catholic faith is all about.

Conversion happened, too, when I was first diagnosed with bladder cancer. I kept thinking 'where did this come from?' In the following weeks and months it was difficult, very very difficult to feel as if things would ever get better. From the initial pain, two trips to the ER, the TURBT and nephrostomy tube they inserted, all through chemotherapy and on into the day I walked into operating room #10 at the Hospital of the University of Pennsylvania in Philadelphia, there was ongoing conversion.

God calls all his faithful through not only His Son but through the Blessed Virgin Mary to live lives of prayer and holiness. Sadly, there are not enough who follow this path in life. As St. John Eudes reminds us, "The Heart of Jesus and Mary is one heart."

If you have trouble relating to a father figure, or find it difficult to talk with Jesus one-on-one, or don't have a clue as to how to pray to the Holy Spirit, turn to Mary. There is no one better to start that conversation with than with a mother. And Mary is mother to all who invoke her name. She can be mother to you, too.

We can place ourselves on the side of Jesus. We can walk the narrow road with Mary. It is easy really. All we need do is to be more prayerful every day; to be more devoted to the Sacred Heart of Jesus and to the Immaculate Heart of Mary. Together these two devotions will help to pull us to Heaven's gate.

In Johnnette Benkovic and Thomas Sullivan's book The Rosary p. 176, there is a beautiful quote:

"on that altar you can place your manger where you too can give Jesus to the world. Or your little part of it. That is all God is really asking of you anyway." Sr. Restituta Kafka

Putting this book together is just my way of saying thanks. I knew that many prayers brought me to a good outcome on the last day of 2018 when the physician's assistant told me there was no further sign of any cancer; not in anything that had been reviewed pathologically.

So, the question became what can I do to say thank you to Jesus and Mary? A 33-day consecration was the answer. Beginning on January 9th and continuing until February 11th, the feast of Our Lady of Lourdes, I undertook the extra prayers and readings, that helped to open my mind to all our faith has waiting for us. There is a treasure here; learn to seek it out.

We can be molded and shaped by Mary to do the work of God. And what is that work in each of our lives? Whatever you are called to do. Whatever small or large endeavor the Lord has mapped out for you. Not all of us are called to be president of the country, or a CEO, or even head of a faculty department.

Some of us do God's work when we offer a helping hand to a neighbor, when we walk into church week after week even when we don't 'feel' holy, when we arise with the sun to start the day all over again. Cooking, driving, going to work, getting children ready for school, tending to an aging parent, paying bills, dusting the furniture, sweeping the floor. Are these things magnificent?

Yes, they are. In the eyes of God, they are as St. Therese would say, our Little Ways. They are not noticed by the world, nor even by our family or friends. They are mostly hidden. They are just the things we do.

My mom was a most extraordinary woman. Don't take my word for it; ask anyone who knew her and they will say the same. Many years ago she worked in a New Jersey shopping mall in one of the big stores, in the jewelry department. Every time she went to work she entered through an employee door. There was usually a guard there and she always said hello to him.

Those were the years of the Cabbage Patch doll craze. Mothers would line up outside of toy stores in the vain effort to procure one of these precious dolls for their kids for Christmas. It just so happened that a shipment of these dolls came into the mall. The mall guard asked my mother if she needed a Cabbage Patch doll or two. He told her he would put them aside for her, because she always spoke to him whenever she came to work, while many other employees walked right on by. He was only a guard, after all.

My mother never expected kindness from this man. She always said hello because it was the right thing to do. The good Lord watches out for us and gives us rewards in the most unexpected ways. Life is in the "little things" we do.

Father Andrew Apostoli was a Franciscan Friar of the Renewal priest. He entered eternal life in December 2017 and was a great advocate of the Holy Spirit. Along with the Third Person of the Trinity, Father had a great devotion to Mary. His fellow priests relate how he would always end his days by reciting his rosary along the stone path at the back of their rectory.

No matter how tired or stressed out he was, he gave Our Lady the last turn of his face, every day. Father believed that when you follow Mary, you will inevitably be led closer to Jesus. It is just her way. He wore out those stones throughout the years, saying his rosary; let us pray with great zeal as he did. Until the stones of life have been made smooth.

Advent is the time when we wait for the Lord. Our unified cry during this prayerful time should be "Come, Lord Jesus." As Mary birthed Jesus, so too, do we get to bring Jesus into the world as well. Especially at Advent.

That quiet season. Where nothing much happens.

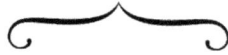

Cardinal Mercier's Prayer to the Holy Spirit

O Holy Spirit

soul of my soul

I adore you.

Enlighten

guide, strengthen and console me.

Tell me what I ought to do

and command me to do it.

I promise to submit to everything

that you ask of me

and to accept all

that you allow to happen to me.

Just show me what is your will.

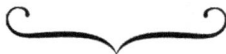

EPILOGUE

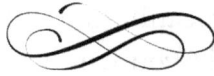

Until and unless you walk through the valley of the shadow of death, called cancer, you will never know the hell it makes of your body. The endless blood taking, CT scans, infusions, hydrations, side effects, the devastating fatigue, doctor visits, and the alone-ness that this illness bestows on you like a gift, you will not understand.

Like I understand. Because we do go through it alone. In your mind and in your heart, you are thoroughly alone. We all climb that mountain when we suffer, but we go on persevering. We go on because we believe that tomorrow will be a better day.

I used to think about how gossamer are the threads of life; how seemingly circumstantial events would line up in my life. I now realize circumstances have nothing to do with it. All truly is in the hand of God. How we find ourselves there, whether we choose to be in that hand, is all up to us.

God gives us problems to catch our attention. Pain, physical or psychological can often overwhelm us. Suddenly we are faced with our own mortality and we don't know what to do. All those things that have composed our lives, don't seem to mean much any longer.

Which is good, because it makes more room for God.

So, how do you have a meaningful Advent? Well, I am hoping if you've read this far, that you will take to heart what has been said here and try, really try, to stay in Advent's moment. Because this season just goes by too fast.

Start Advent traditions if you don't already do them. They are something of value to pass on to your children. This is the time when we prepare for Christ's coming; and it's specially built in to these four weeks leading up to Christmas Day. Here are a few suggestions for you:

Advent Wreath. For sure, have an Advent wreath. There are supplies you can buy at any craft store and have your children help you to fashion the wreath just right. You can buy Advent candles in any big box store or online. Just do it.

Advent Calendar. My Advent calendar is almost as old as me. It was my mom's when I was growing up and it came with a poem; each stanza was a clue to which window or door to open. I no longer have the poem, but the memories have never faded. Every year my Advent calendar is the first part of my Christmas decorations to be put out.

Nativity Scenes. Put out the manger and put the baby Jesus someplace far away from it, somewhere in your home. Then day by day, bring Him a little closer to where he will be laying on Christmas Day. It's so much more fulfilling than that elf on a shelf.

Advent Prayers. This season has many beautiful devotional books that will take you deeper into the very meaning of what Advent brings to each one of us. Prepare yourself spiritually by reading every day why it is that Jesus came to us as an infant. The King of Kings was never expected in this way.

Special Prayers. During Advent it is so nice to concentrate on the Joyful Mysteries every day. Saying a special rosary daily with intentions that come from your heart will surely make Mary and her Son very happy.

Then there are the 'O Antiphons'. These begin on December 17 and lead us right up until Christmas Eve. Here you will find some of the most beautiful titles that herald the coming of the Son of God. In 2018, I completely missed the O Antiphons; my surgery took place that day and for the next week I wasn't in very good shape for much of anything.

Advent Music. Find and download beautiful sounds of the Advent season. Play Advent CD's as well as traditional Christmas songs. These will prepare your heart for Jesus and make it specially soft and welcoming for Him.

Total Consecration to Jesus Through Mary. This is known as a 33-day consecration that anyone can do anytime of the year. If you start on November 29th, you may already be in the season of Advent, or on the very cusp of this special time in the church. Your consecration date will end on January 1, which is not just New Year's Day, but the feast of the Solemnity of Mary, Mother of God. What better way to begin the year!

Using the format put forth by St. Louis de Montfort, you will go deep into readings and prayers for 33 days. St. Louis tells us that Jesus came into the world through Mary and for all of us to ever be close to our Lord, we should always go through Mary. This is the most beautiful devotion I can recommend to you and you can do a 33-day consecration every year. Daily, you can consecrate your day to Our Mother and she will take your petitions to Jesus. You will only increase your love for Jesus and Mary through a consecration and what better time than Advent to begin!

The theme of Advent then is one of longing. We yearn for something more – after all, 'our hearts are restless until they rest in thee', as St. Augustine reminds us. Yet, we are told to be on the lookout for Christ. Prepare yourself. Stay awake. Walk through this beautiful and holy season with Mary.

There are those who will tell you that reciting the Hail Mary incessantly is not fruitful prayer. If said correctly, there is no more productive prayer this side of heaven. As found in True Devotion to Mary by St. Louis de Montfort: "They tell us that the Hail Mary is a heavenly dew for watering the earth, which is the soul, to make it bring forth its fruit in season; and that a soul which is not watered by that prayer bears no fruit, and brings forth only thorns and brambles, and is ready to be cursed. (Heb. 6:8)."

It is Mary who will help us to prepare ourselves. With her aid, we will be made ready to birth Jesus Christ into our world, right where we are, to the people we know in the here and now. When Christmas Day is at last upon us we will really mean it when we say "Merry Christmas!" – because Christmas, the Christ-child, will really be born in us for all to see.

So, for now, I am back to walking my dogs, babysitting my grand daughters, driving to stores, making my spaghetti sauce and knitting to my hearts' content. My doctors have told me I am 'cancer-free' and I am so grateful for these words. Summer is here, and a complete year has rolled around since that fateful July day. Every day brings with it a renewal of the earth. Please God, let there be a renewal of my mind as well.

"To whom much is given, much will be required." (Luke 12:48) We have been given the truth of our Catholic faith through Jesus Christ our Lord and we have been given His most Blessed Mother. How happy we should be. If we steep ourselves in every season of the Church year, we will become the people God yearns for us to be.

I always keep in mind that I didn't suffer alone. I had my family always asking how I was, and in the background at all times, was Our Lady and Jesus. Our Lord suffered greatly for us. That is why if we have to suffer a little bit in this life, then we do what has been ordained for us. We are never alone in our sufferings.

It is not just ourselves that desire and long to get to Heaven. We can also help those around us to follow that path with us. Dusty, thorny, narrow and unknown is the path before us. However, we don't travel alone – for we have the best of company.

The Blessed Mother and her Son.

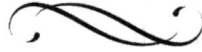

You know I just couldn't close without saying a word about my husband Bob. He was my life-line during all those months where sometimes it was hard to even remember what the day of the week was. He did all the housecleaning, laundry, food shopping and taking the dogs out, all day long. He would get me anything I wanted, juice, tea or soup, whenever I asked him. Many was the time he had just sat down and I would request something of him again. On those days where I was too sick to stay home alone, he would stay with me and forego his four-day-a-week job so I wouldn't be by myself.

He did everything for me and when I would crawl into bed at 8 p.m. every night he would make sure I was as comfortable as I could be and then he would kiss me goodnight. I do not know how anyone could get through cancer treatments on their own. Thank God it wasn't in the cards that way for me.

I was reminded of the movie Watch On The Rhine starring Bette Davis and Paul Lukas from 1943. Towards the end of the film they must part because he has to return to Germany and almost certain death. Just before they part, Bette Davis tells Paul Lukas,

"I have loved just once and for all my life."

Bob and I met on June 27, 1970. I was 18 years old, he was 19. That's a long time ago. That day is the feast day of Our Lady of Perpetual Help, my very favorite image of Mary and Jesus out of all the thousands of images there are of the two of them. We have been married since October 22, 1972, another feast day, that of St. John Paul II. That also, is a long time ago. During our wedding ceremony, we laid a bouquet of flowers on Mary's altar as a tribute to Our Lady. I believe Mary has been in our lives ever since. We've had our ups and downs, our shout-fests, arguments, and times when we seemed to be a million miles apart.

Through it all we've also had our faith. Our Catholic faith. There is nothing quite like it in the world. Or on this earth.

In my many readings that I did when writing this book, I was particularly struck by one little story told by Fr. Andrew Apostoli, a Franciscan Friar of the Renewal. Years ago while attending an exhibit at the Metropolitan Museum of Art in NYC, Father encountered a poor, homeless man sitting on the steps leading into the building. "Are you for real, or part of the show?" the man asked Fr. Andrew.

That is the question we should be asking ourselves every day. Do we go along to get along, do we agree with everything that is thrust into our faces, even when we sense wrongdoing, do we live our lives on the surface, enjoying what is there but yearning for something deeper?

Pray, pray very much. These are the words of Our Lady at Fatima.

When the whole world seems to be going down the drain, take out your rosary and pray. Delve deeply into the mysteries of God. Find, through the Holy Spirit, that which he is asking of you. There is nothing in this world more rewarding or more fulfilling.

Your Advent and your life will be transformed.

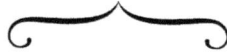

The Hail Mary

Ave Maria,

gratia plena,

Dominus tecum.

Benedicta tu in mulieribus,

et benedictus fructus ventris tui,

Jesus.

Sancta Maria, Mater Dei,

ora pro nobis peccatoribus,

nunc in hora mortis nostrae.

~ Amen.~

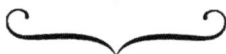

Book List

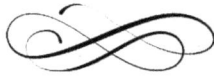

Here is a Book List which includes my favorite titles:

Advent With Our Lady of Fatima
– Donna Marie Cooper O'Boyle

Aim Higher!
Spiritual and Marian Reflections of St. Maximilian Kolbe
– Fr. Dominic Wisz, OFM Conv.

Ignatius The Holy Bible, Catholic Edition

Immaculate Conception and the Holy Spirit
The Marian Teachings of St. Maximilian Kolbe
– Fr. H.M. Manteau-Bonamy, OP

Life of Union With Mary
– Fr. Emile Neubert

The Rosary Your Weapon for Spiritual Warfare
– Johnnette Benkovic & Thomas K. Sullivan

**The Secrets, Chastisement, and Triumph
Of the Two Hearts of Jesus and Mary**
– Kelly Bowring

The World's First Love, Mary Mother of God
– Fulton J. Sheen

True Devotion to Mary
– St. Louis de Montfort

United States Grace Force Prayer Book
– Fr. Richard M. Heilman

Virtuous Leadership An Agenda for Personal Excellence
– Alexandre Havard

Waiting for Christ Meditations for Advent and Christmas
– St. John Henry Newman

With Mary to Jesus
– Rev. Joseph M. Esper

www.ingramcontent.com/pod-product-compliance
Lightning Source LLC
Chambersburg PA
CBHW060517280326
41933CB00014B/2995